Copyright 2023

Table of Contents

The Mediterranean diet is based on the diets of people from Crete, Greece, and Southern Italy. The Mediterranean diet has become popular because individuals show low rate of heart disease, chronic disease, and obesity. The Mediterranean diet profile focuses on whole grains, good fats (fish, olive oil, nuts etc.), vegetables, fruits, fish, and very low consumption of any non-fish meat. Along with food, the Mediterranean diet emphasizes the need to spend time eating with family and physical activity.

BREAKFAST

1. Thousand Island Dressing

Prep Time: 5 Minutes

Cook Time: 00 minutes

Servings: 14

Ingredients

- 1 cup mayonnaise
- 1/4 cup ketchup
- 1/3 cup sweet relish
- ½ teaspoon sweet paprika
- 2 tablespoons fresh lemon juice (from 1 lemon)
- 1 tablespoon grated onion
- 1 clove garlic, minced
- ½ teaspoon kosher salt
- ¼ teaspoon freshly cracked black pepper

Instructions

1. In a small bowl, whisk together the mayonnaise, ketchup, relish, paprika, lemon juice, onion, garlic, salt and pepper, until combined. Store refrigerated in an airtight container for up to 1 week.
2. Yield: 1 ¾ cups

Prep Time: 10 Minutes

Cook Time: 20 minutes

Servings: 6

Ingredients

- 8 large eggs
- ⅓ cup heavy cream, half-and-half, or whole milk
- 4 ounces crumbled or 1 cup of shredded cheese
- 2 tablespoons chopped fresh herbs, plus more for serving
- 1 teaspoon sea salt
- ½ teaspoon freshly cracked black pepper
- 2 tablespoons extra-virgin olive oil
- 3 cups diced vegetables
- 1 garlic clove, minced (optional)
- 2 cups loosely packed, roughly chopped greens
- 5-7 slices cooked bacon, crumbled
- Flaky salt, for serving

Instructions

1. Preheat the oven to 400°F with a rack in the center position.

2. In a large bowl, beat the eggs. Add the cream, 3/4 cup of the cheese, the herbs, salt, and pepper. Stir to combine.

3. Heat the olive oil in a 10-inch, ovenproof skillet over medium-heat. Once the oil is glistening, add the vegetables and cook until softened, 6-8 minutes. Add the garlic and cook until fragrant, about 1 minute more. Add the greens and cook, stirring, until wilted, about 4 minutes. Stir in the crumbled bacon.

4. Pour the egg mixture over the vegetable mixture and give it a quick stir to incorporate the eggs and filling evenly. Cook, undisturbed, until the edges are set, about 2 minutes. Top the frittata with the remaining ¼ cup cheese and transfer the skillet to the oven and bake until the eggs are set, about 12-14 minutes. The eggs should barely move when you jiggle the pan.

5. Top the frittata with the extra herbs. Slice into wedges. Sprinkle with flaky salt to taste, and then serve.

Prep Time: 15 Minutes

Cook Time: 1hr 30 minutes

Servings: 8

Ingredients

For the Prime Rib:

- 5-6 pounds bone-in rib roast
- 4 tablespoons coarse sea salt
- 3 tablespoons freshly cracked black pepper
- 1 teaspoon garlic powder
- 1 teaspoon mustard powder
- 1 teaspoon minced fresh thyme
- 1 (1.1 ounce) Pack Johnny's French Dip Au Jus seasoning
- 2 heads garlic
- 2 tablespoon extra-virgin olive oil
- For the Horseradish Sauce
- ½ cup heavy whipping cream, chilled
- ½ cup sour cream
- ¼ cup mayonnaise

- 3-6 tablespoons horseradish sauce
- 2 tablespoons minced chives
- ½ teaspoon sea salt

Instructions

1. Make the prime rib. Line a baking dish with paper towels 24 hours before roasting, place the rib roast in the prepared baking dish. Rub the rib roast all over with the salt. Chill in the refrigerator, uncovered, for 24 hours.
2. Make the horseradish sauce. In a small bowl, whisk the heavy cream until soft peaks form. Carefully fold in the sour cream, mayonnaise, horseradish sauce, chives and salt. Cover and place in the refrigerator until ready to use. Store refrigerated in an airtight container for up to one week.
3. Prepare the rib roast (2 hours before roasting). In a small bowl, combine the pepper, garlic powder, mustard powder, thyme, and ½ of the Au Jus powder. Rub the roast all over with the spice mixture. Rest uncovered until the prime rib roast has come to room temperature, about 2 hours.
4. Preheat the oven to 450°F.

5. Place the roast, with bones on the bottom, in a roasting pan or large ovenproof skillet. Trim the tops off the garlic heads just enough to expose the cloves. Place each head on a separate piece of aluminum foil. Pour the olive oil over the exposed cloves. Wrap the foil around each head of garlic and place them in the roasting pan with the prime rib roast. Roast for 20 minutes, then reduce the temperature to 325°F and roast until desired doneness is achieved on an instant read thermometer, 60-70 minutes (see Note). Remove the roast and the garlic from the oven and rest for 20 minutes.

6. Transfer the roast to a carving board, place the roasting pan on the stove top and bring the dripping to a boil over high heat, add the remaining au jus seasoning powder and 1 cup of water, whisking vigorously until reduced by half, about 6 minutes. Transfer to a serving vessel.

7. Using a sharp knife, thinly slice the meat and serve. Serve with horseradish cream, roasted garlic (squeezed from their skins), and au jus sauce alongside.

8. Note: The most precise way to measure the doneness of prime rib is with an instant-read thermometer. For rare cook until the internal doneness is 125°F;

medium-rare 135°F; medium 145°F; medium- well 150°F; and well 160°F. Roast to your preference, but prime rib is traditionally served rare!v

Prep Time: 30 Minutes

Cook Time: 1hr 10 minutes

Servings: 8

Ingredients

- 2 large eggplants, cut into ¼-inch-thick slices
- 3 teaspoons kosher salt
- ½ cup all-purpose flour
- 4 large eggs
- 3½ cups panko breadcrumbs
- 1½ teaspoons garlic powder
- 1½ teaspoons onion powder
- 2 teaspoons Italian seasoning
- 2 tablespoons extra-virgin olive oil
- 3 cups marinara sauce
- 16 ounces fresh mozzarella, thinly sliced, we like buffalo mozzarella
- 8 ounces freshly grated Parmesan cheese

Instructions

1. Preheat the oven to 400°F. Line 2 sheet pans with parchment paper.

2. Arrange eggplant slices on the prepared baking sheet and sprinkle with 1½ teaspoons of the salt. Set aside for 10 minutes. Pat dry with a paper towel.

3. Place the flour in a shallow bowl or pie pan. In a separate shallow bowl, beat the eggs. Place the panko, garlic powder, onion powder, Italian seasoning, and remaining 1 teaspoon of salt in a third shallow bowl. Dip each eggplant slice into the flour, then into the beaten egg, allowing the excess to drip off. Press each slice into the panko mixture to coat and return to the sheet pans. Drizzle the slices with olive oil.

4. Bake the eggplant for 30 minutes, rotating the baking sheets halfway through, or until golden. Reduce heat to 375°F.

5. Add ¼ cup of the marinara sauce to a 9x13-inch baking dish. Spread out into an even layer. Transfer half of the eggplant slices to the sauce in an even layer, slightly overlapping if needed. Cover the eggplant with ½ of the remaining marinara sauce. Top with half of the mozzarella slices and half of the Parmesan. Repeat with remaining ingredients, finishing with the Parmesan.

Bake until the cheese is golden brown, about 35-40 minutes.

6. Serve immediately.

Prep Time: 10 Minutes

Cook Time: 15 minutes

Servings: 4

Ingredients

- 12 ounces orecchiette pasta
- ¾ pound mild Italian sausage, ground or casing removed
- 6 garlic cloves, thinly sliced
- 1 cup heavy cream
- 1 cup freshly grated parmesan cheese, plus more for serving
- Sea salt, for serving
- Freshly cracked black pepper, for serving
- 2 teaspoons fresh lemon juice (from 1 lemon)
- 1 bunch Tuscan or Lacinato kale, tough stems discarded and leaves roughly chopped (about 4 cups)
- Red pepper flakes, for serving (optional)

Instructions

1. Bring a large pot of salted water to a boil over high heat.
   Cook the pasta until al dente, according to the package
   directions. Drain and set aside.

2. Meanwhile, heat a large nonstick saucepan over
   medium heat. Add the sausage and cook, breaking it up
   with a wooden spoon, until browned, about 8 minutes.
   Add the garlic and cook until fragrant, 1 more minutes.
   Using a slotted spoon, transfer the sausage and garlic
   to a bowl.

3. Add the cream and parmesan to the saucepan. Cook,
   stirring often, until thick enough to coat the back of a
   wooden spoon, about 5 minutes. Add salt and pepper
   to taste. Add the lemon juice and kale and cook, stirring
   occasionally, until wilted, about 2 minutes.

4. Return the sausage mixture to the saucepan along with
   the drained pasta, stir to combine.

5. To serve, sprinkle the pasta with parmesan and red
   pepper flakes, if using.

Prep Time: 5 Minutes

Cook Time: 20 minutes

Servings: 4

Ingredients

- 2 large fennel bulbs
- 2 tablespoons extra-virgin olive oil
- ½ teaspoon garlic powder
- 1 teaspoon kosher salt
- Freshly cracked black pepper, to taste

Instructions

1. Preheat the oven to 425°F.
2. Trim the stalks and flat root base away from the fennel bulbs, reserve the fronds for garnish. Halve and cut into ⅓-inch wedges.
3. Spread the wedges out on a large rimmed baking sheet and toss with the olive oil, garlic powder, and salt.

4. Roast the fennel until tender and beginning to brown, about 20 minutes. Turn on the broiler and cook for another 2 minutes, until the edges are caramelized.

Prep Time: 20 Minutes

Cook Time: 30 minutes

Servings: 4

Ingredients

- 2 teaspoons light brown sugar
- 1 ½ teaspoons sea salt or celery salt
- 1 ½ teaspoons garlic powder
- ¼ teaspoon freshly cracked black pepper
- ¾ teaspoon paprika
- 3 large russet potatoes (about 2 ¼ pounds), scrubbed and cut into 1 ½ -inch-thick wedges
- 1/4 cup extra-virgin olive oil
- Ranch dressing, store-bought or homemade, for serving

Instructions

1. Preheat the oven to 450°F. With a rack in the center position. Line a rimmed sheet pan with parchment paper.

2. In a small bowl, combine the brown sugar, salt, garlic powder, pepper, and paprika. Place the potatoes on the prepared sheet pan and drizzle them with the olive oil. Sprinkle on the spice mixture, toss to coat, and spread potatoes into an even layer. Bake until golden brown, about 30 minutes.

3. Serve with ranch.

Prep Time: 5 Minutes

Cook Time: 5 minutes

Servings: 8

Ingredients

- 1/2 cup buttermilk
- 1/2 cup mayonnaise
- 1/2 cup sour cream
- 1 tsp dried parsley (or 2 tsp fresh)
- 1 tsp onion powder
- 1 tsp garlic powder
- 1 tsp dried dill
- 1/2 tsp salt

Instructions

2. In a small bowl whisk together all ingredients until smooth. Can be stored in refrigerator in an airtight container for up to 2 weeks.

Prep Time: 30 Minutes

Cook Time: 50 minutes

Servings: 8

Ingredients

For the Potatoes:

- 4 teaspoons kosher salt
- 3 pounds russet potatoes, peeled and cut into 2-inch cubes
- 1 cup (2 sticks) unsalted butter, softened
- 1 cup whole milk
- 1 teaspoon garlic powder
- ½ teaspoon freshly cracked black pepper

For the filling:

- 2 tablespoons extra-virgin olive oil
- 2 pounds 90/10 ground beef or ground lamb
- 1 ½ teaspoons kosher salt
- 1 cup finely chopped onion
- 2 large carrots, peeled and finely diced
- 1 cup finely chopped fennel

- 2 garlic cloves, minced
- 2 tablespoons all-purpose or gluten-free flour
- 2 tablespoons tomato paste
- 2 cups beef broth or stock
- ½ teaspoon freshly cracked black pepper, plus more for serving
- 1 teaspoon finely chopped fresh thyme, plus more for serving
- 1 teaspoon finely chopped fresh rosemary
- 1 cup frozen peas

Instructions

3. Preheat the oven to 400°F with a rack in the center position.
4. Fill a large pot with water and 3 teaspoons of the salt. Add the potatoes and bring to a boil over high heat. Cook until fork tender, about 15 minutes. Drain and set aside.
5. In the same pot, combine the butter and milk over medium-low heat. Cook, stirring, until the butter is melted, about 2 minutes. Using a potato ricer, rice the potatoes over the hot butter mixture. (Alternatively, mash the potatoes directly into the liquid, taking care

not to overwork them.) Season with the garlic powder, pepper and the remaining 1 teaspoon salt.

6. Heat 1 tablespoon of the olive oil in a large skillet over medium-high heat. Once the oil is glistening, add the ground beef and season with 1 teaspoon of the salt. Cook, undisturbed, until browned, about 5 minutes. Using a wooden spoon, break up the meat and continue cooking until cooked through, about 5 minutes more. Drain any excess grease and transfer to a plate.

7. Reduce the heat under the same skillet to medium and add remaining tablespoon of olive oil, onions, carrots, and fennel. Season with remaining ½ teaspoon of salt and cook, stirring often, until vegetables are softened, about 5-7 minutes. Add the garlic and cook until fragrant, about 2 more minutes more.

8. Add the flour and tomato paste and cook, stirring continuously, until tomato paste has darkened, about 1 minute. Slowly stir in beef stock, pepper, thyme, and rosemary and bring to a simmer. Add the browned beef and any collected juices and frozen peas and simmer, stirring occasionally until sauce has thickened and liquid is mostly absorbed, about 10 minutes.

9. Transfer the filling to a 9x13-inch baking dish and spread out evenly. Top with mashed potatoes, and

smooth out into an even layer using the back of a spoon. Bake until the filling is bubbling and potatoes are golden brown, about 20 minutes.

10. Top with freshly cracked pepper and fresh thyme and let cool for 15 minutes before serving.

Prep Time: 5 Minutes

Cook Time: 30 minutes

Servings: 4

Ingredients

For the Béchamel sauce:

- 3 tablespoons salted butter
- 1 1/2 tablespoons all-purpose flour
- 1 cup whole milk
- 2 to 3 sprigs fresh thyme, plus more for serving
- 1 tablespoon Dijon mustard
- 1/4 teaspoon kosher salt
- 1/8 teaspoon ground nutmeg
- For the for the sandwiches
- 8 tablespoons (1 stick) salted butter, softened
- 8 thick slices white sandwich bread
- 12 slices deli ham
- 2 cups grated Gruyère cheese

For serving:

- 2 teaspoons chopped fresh chives, optional

- Freshly cracked black pepper

Instructions

1. Preheat the oven to 375°F with a rack in the center position.

2. Make the béchamel sauce. Add the butter to a medium saucepan over medium heat and whisk until melted. Sprinkle in the flour and cook, whisking continuously, until the mixture is combined and the butter begins to bubble, about 30 seconds. Slowly whisk in the milk until smooth. Add the thyme and cook, whisking, until the sauce thickens, about 2 minutes more. Whisk in the mustard, salt, and nutmeg, then remove from heat and discard thyme stems.

3. Make the sandwiches. Spread 1 tablespoon butter onto one side of each of the bread slices. Place four of the bread slices butter-sides down on a sheet pan. Place three folded slices of ham on each, and top each with 1/4 cup grated cheese. Top with the remaining slices of bread, butter-sides up.

4. Bake until bread is golden brown and cheese has melted, about 6 minutes. Remove from the oven, flip,

and repeat on the other side. Remove the sheet pan from the oven and turn on the broiler.

5. Evenly pour the béchamel sauce over the sandwiches, then top with the remaining cheese (about ¼ cup per sandwich). Broil until the cheese is bubbling and beginning to brown, 3 to 4 minutes.

6. Sprinkle the sandwiches with chives, fresh thyme, and black pepper, if desired. Serve warm.

11. Easy Chicken Ramen Soup

Prep Time: 15 Minutes

Cook Time: 15 minutes

Servings: 2

Ingredients

- 1 tbsp Organic Sesame Oil
- 4 garlic cloves, minced
- 2 tbsp ginger, minced
- 6 cups chicken stock
- 3 tbsp soy sauce
- 1/2 bunch green onions, chopped
- oz package shiitake mushrooms, sliced
- 1 cup cooked chicken, shredded or sliced
- 1/2 tsp salt
- 3 packs ramen noodles (flavor packet discarded)
- 2 6 minute eggs
- sesame seeds
- Scallion Chili Sesame Oil
- 1/4 cup Organic Sesame Oil

- 1 tbsp chili paste/ sauce
- 1/2 bunch green onions, chopped

Instructions

1. In a small bowl, combine the 3 ingredients for the Scallion, Chili, Sesame oil. Set aside.
2. Heat 1 tablespoon Organic Sesame Oil in a medium sized soup pot. Add the garlic and ginger and sauté until fragrant.
3. Add the chicken stock, soy sauce, green onions, mushrooms, chicken and salt and bring to a boil. Add the 3 packages of ramen (noodles only, discard the flavor packet). Boil for 2 minutes until noodles are soft. Remove from heat.
4. Sprinkle the sesame seeds over the soup and place the soft boiled (6 minute) egg in the bowl. Serve with the Scallion, chili, and sesame oil.

Prep Time: 20 Minutes

Cook Time: 40 minutes

Servings: 8

Ingredients

- Meatballs
- 1 lbground beef
- 1 lb ground pork
- ¼ cup flat leaf parsley, minced
- ½ tsp ground allspice
- ½ tsp ground nutmeg
- ¾ cup yellow onion, grated (about 1 medium onion)
- 2 tsp salt
- ½ tsp pepper, freshly ground
- 4 cloves garlic, minced
- ¾ cup panko
- 2 eggs
- 2 tbsp olive oil
- Cream Gravy
- ½ cup butter
- ½ cup flour

- 4 cups beef broth
- 1 tsp salt
- ¼ tsp pepper
- 1 tbsp lemon juice
- ¼ tsp ground allspice
- ¼ tsp ground nutmeg
- 1 cup heavy cream

Instructions

1. In a large bowl, mix the beef, pork, parsley, allspice, nutmeg, grated onion, salt, pepper, garlic, panko and eggs until combined.
2. Using a tablespoon or cookie scoop, measure out the meat mixture into roughly 35 (1.5 inch) balls.
3. In a large pan, heat 2 tablespoon of olive oil over medium-high heat. Add ½ of the meatballs and cook until browned on all sides. This takes about 5 minutes. Set aside
4. When all of the meatballs are browned, pour off any excess grease in the pan, into a heatproof vessel. Lower the heat to medium and add the butter to the pan. When the butter begins to bubble, sprinkle in the flour

and cook for 1 minute. Add the beef broth to the pan a little at a time.

5. Whisk the gravy until the broth is all incorporated. Add salt, pepper, lemon juice, allspice and nutmeg. Whisk a few more times. Slowly add the cream.

6. Once the gravy begins to simmer, add the meatballs back into the pan.

7. Simmer until the gravy has thicken up a bit and the meatballs are cooked all the way through, about 8-10 minutes.

8. Serve warm over mashed potatoes or egg noodles, alongside steamed veggies and lingonberry jam.

Cooking Notes:

1. Gluten Free Version: if you want to keep this recipe gluten free, you can sub the breadcrumbs for a gluten-free version. To keep the gluten out of the gravy, you will want to reserve 1 cup of beef stock and mix it with ⅓ cup corn starch. Add it to the gravy at the end to thicken it up.

2. I like to shape the meatballs and place them on a piece of parchment paper for easy clean up and less dishes. Then I use another piece of parchment to place the browned meatballs on, again, easy clean up, less dishes.

3. If you take your time adding the beef broth, your gravy
    will stay thick, taking less time overall.

4. Take care not to boil the cream. It might separate if you
    do. Keep it at a simmer until the meatballs are cooked
    all the way through.

5. The meatballs should reach an internal temperature of
    165° F and no longer be pink on the inside.

Prep Time: 25 Minutes

Cook Time: 25 minutes

Servings: 4

Ingredient

- Lemon Parmesan Rice
- 1 ½ cups long grain white or jasmine rice, rinsed under cold water
- 2 ½ cups chicken broth
- ½ teaspoon garlic powder
- zest and juice of 1 lemon
- 4 tablespoons salted butter
- ½ cup grated parmesan cheese
- sea salt and freshly cracked black pepper to taste
- ¼ cup capers, drained, optional
- Skillet-Fried Pork Cutlets
- 3 (1-inch thick) boneless pork chops (about 1 pound total)
- 1 teaspoon kosher salt
- ¼ teaspoon freshly cracked black pepper
- 2 large eggs

- 1 ¼ cups panko

- 3 tablespoons vegetable oil

- Creamy Lemon Dressing

- 2 teaspoons lemon zest

- 2 tablespoons lemon juice, from 1 large lemon

- 1 teaspoons granulated sugar

- 1 clove garlic, minced

- ¼ teaspoon sea salt

- ½ teaspoon raw apple cider vinegar

- ¼ cup mayonnaise

- 2 tablespoons extra-virgin olive oil

For Serving:

- lemon wedges

- arugula

- cherry tomatoes, cut in half

Instructions

1. Make the rice. To a medium saucepan add the rice, chicken broth, garlic powder, lemon zest and juice, along with 2 tablespoons of the butter, stir to combine.

2. Turn the heat to high, cook, stirring, until the liquid begins to boil. Cover with a tight fitting lid, turn the

heat to low and simmer until tender and all of the liquid is absorbed, about 18 minutes.

3. Stir in the remaining 2 tablespoons butter, parmesan cheese, salt and pepper to taste and capers, if using.

4. While the rice is cooking, make the pork. Place 1 pork chop between 2 sheets of parchment paper or plastic wrap. Using a meat mallet or rolling pin, pound to ¼-inch thickness. Repeat with remaining pork chops. Season on both sides with the salt and pepper.

5. In a shallow bowl or pie pan, beat the eggs. Place the panko in a separate shallow bowl. Dip each pork chop into the egg, allowing the excess to drip off. Press each pork chop into the panko to coat evenly.

6. Heat 2 tablespoons of the vegetable oil in a large skillet, over medium-high heat. Once the oil is glistening, add 2 pork chops and cook, undisturbed, until golden brown, about 3 to 4 minutes. Flip the pork chops and cook, undisturbed until golden brown on both sides, another 3 to 4 minutes. Transfer the pork to a cutting board. Add the remaining 1 tablespoon oil to the skillet and repeat with the remaining pork chops. Let the pork chops rest for 5 minutes before slicing.

7. Make the dressing. To a jar with a tight fitting lid, add the lemon zest, lemon juice, sugar, garlic, minced, salt,

vinegar, mayonnaise, olive oil. Place the lid on and shake until combined, about 30 seconds. Alternatively you can add all of the ingredients to a bowl and whisk until combined.

8. Divide the rice into 4 bowls. Top with sliced pork, arugula, and tomatoes. Drizzle with dressing and an extra squeeze of lemon juice if desired.

Prep Time: 15 Minutes

Cook Time: 10 minutes

Servings: 4

Ingredients

- 4 slices of artisan bread, cut 1 inch in thickness
- 1 lb cooked shrimp, roughly chopped1/3 cup good mayonnaise
- 1 tbsp fresh squeezed lemon juice
- 1 tsp worcestershire
- 2 tsp Old Bay Seasoning
- 3 tbsp celery, minced
- 1 tbsp shallot, finely copped
- 2 tbsp capers
- 8 slices of tomato
- 1 cup sharp cheddar cheese, grated

Instructions

1. In a medium sized bowl, whisk mayonnaise, lemon juice, old bay seasoning, Worcestershire, capers,

shallots and celery. Fold shrimp into mayonnaise mixture and toss just enough to ensure it is evenly coated.

2. Place sliced bread on a baking sheet. Broil the bread on low just long enough to get a slight crisp on the top side, about 2 minutes. Flip bread over and toast the other side for another 2 minutes. Once both sides are lightly toasted, remove them from the oven.

3. Divide the shrimp mixture evenly among the toast. Top with 2 slices of tomato each and cover in shredded sharp cheddar. Place back under the broiler until the cheese melted and beginning to brown in spots. Serve immediately.

Prep Time: 25 Minutes

Cook Time: 20 minutes

Servings: 6

Ingredients

- 1 1/2 lbs asparagus, woody ends trimmed off
- 3 tbsp butter, divided
- 2 tbsp flour
- 1 cup whole milk
- 1 tbsp whole grain mustard
- 1/2 tsp salt
- 1/2 tsp freshly ground pepper
- 1/4 tsp nutmeg
- 1/2 cup parmesan cheese, grated
- 3/4 cup Gruyère, grated
- 3/4 cup panko bread crumbs
- 1 tbsp flat leaf parsley, minced, optional

Instructions

1. Heat oven to 400° F.

2. Bring salted water (1 tbsp salt for every 4 quarts water) to a boil in a large pot. Blanch asparagus in the boiling water for 4 minutes. Asparagus should be tender, but still crisp. Drain asparagus, transfer to a gratin or other baking dish, set aside.

3. In a small saucepan or skillet, melt 2 tablespoons butter over medium heat until bubbly. When the foam subsides, add the flour and whisk until thickened and fragrant, 1 minute.

4. Slowly add the milk to the butter mixture and whisk for 2 minutes until slightly thickened.

5. Season the sauce by adding the mustard, salt, pepper and nutmeg. Whisk until fully incorporated. Add the parmesan cheese, stir until combined.

6. Pour the sauce over the asparagus in the baking dish. Sprinkle gruyere over the sauce.

7. Bake in the hot oven until bubbly and beginning to brown. 15-20 minutes.

8. While the gratin is baking, toast the panko along with the remaining tablespoon of butter, in a small skillet over medium heat. Stir continually until the panko is a nice golden brown. Set aside.

9. When gratin comes out of the oven, sprinkle with toasted panko and parsley and a little extra parmesan cheese. Serve warm. Enjoy.

Prep Time: 20 Minutes

Cook Time: 15 minutes

Servings: 6

Ingredients

- 1 lb store-bought or homemade pizza dough
- 1 (14 oz) jar pizza sauce
- 10-12 oz mozzarella cheese, shredded
- 15-20 salami slices
- 1/4 medium red onion, sliced very thin
- 1 jalapeño, seeded, thinly sliced
- 1/2 cup castelvetrano olives, pitted, sliced in half
- olive oil, for brushing edges and pizza pan
- everything Bagel Seasoning, recipe below
- 1/4 cup honey
- red pepper flakes, optional
- Everything Bagel Seasoning
- 2 tsp poppy seeds
- 2 tsp onion flakes
- 2 tsp garlic flakes
- 2 tsp sesame seeds

- 1/2 tsp coarse salt

Instructions

1. Heat oven to 500° F. Or as high as your oven will go.
2. To make the everything bagel seasoning, mix all ingredients in a small bowl, set aside.
3. Let the pizza dough come to room temperature for 30 minutes before stretching or rolling out onto a lightly floured surface with a rolling pin.
4. When your dough is roughly 10 inches in diameter or ½ inch thick, place it on lightly oiled parchment paper on top of a baking sheet or sprinkled underneath with corn meal to prevent sticking, pizza pan, or pre-heated pizza stone.
5. Spoon pizza sauce (to desired thin or thickness) onto dough leaving 1-inch of crust exposed around the edges. Cover the sauce with ¾ of the mozzarella cheese.
6. Place the salami, onion, jalapeños, and olives onto the pizza. Sprinkle with remaining cheese.
7. Brush edges of pizza with olive oil and sprinkle with the everything bagel seasoning.

8. Place pizza in the oven for 10-12 minutes until edges
   are golden brown and the center of the crust is crispy.

9. Remove from oven, drizzle with honey and sprinkle
   with red pepper flakes. Serve with extra honey for
   dipping the crust into.

Prep Time: 30 Minutes

Cook Time: 15 minutes

Servings: 10

Ingredients

Beef Patties:

- 1 pound 80/20 ground beef
- 2 garlic cloves, minced
- 3 ounces blue cheese, crumbled
- 1 tablespoon Worcestershire
- 1 tablespoon Dijon mustard
- 1 teaspoon sea salt
- 2 teaspoon freshly cracked black pepper
- 3 tablespoons extra-virgin olive oil

Sun-Dried Tomato Mayo:

- 1 cup mayonnaise
- 1 tablespoon lemon zest
- 1 tablespoon lemon juice
- 1/2 cup oil packed sun-dried tomatoes, drained, roughly chopped

- 2 tablespoons finely chopped chives
- 2 garlic cloves, mined
- ½ teaspoon freshly cracked black pepper

For Serving:

- 10 mini brioche buns
- Sweet and spicy pickles (or store bought)
- Arugula
- Toothpicks (optional)

Instructions

1. Make the sun-dried tomato mayo. In a small bowl stir together the mayonnaise, lemon zest, lemon juice, sun-dried tomatoes, chives, and garlic and pepper until combined. Can be made ahead and stored in an airtight container in the refrigerator for up to 2 weeks.
2. Make the beef patties. In a large bowl, combine the beef, garlic, blue cheese, Worcestershire, Dijon, salt and pepper. Using your hands form 10 patties 2-inches in diameter and ½ inch thick. Using your thumb make a small indentation in the middle of each patty.
3. Heat the 2 tablespoons of the olive oil in a large cast iron skillet over medium-high heat. Once the oil is

smoking, arrange half of the patties in the skillet. Cook undisturbed until browned, about 3 minutes. Flip the patties over and cook until browned, 2 more minutes. Continue flipping until desired doneness is achieved. Transfer the patties to a paper towel lined plate. Repeat with remaining patties.

4. Meanwhile toast the buns. Place the buns cut side up on a baking sheet and broil 2-3 minutes until golden brown.

5. Serve the beef patties on the buns alongside spicy pickles, arugula and sun-dried tomato mayo. Use a toothpick to hold together, if desired.

6. Note: Rare 120°-125°, med-rare 130°-135°, medium 140°-145°, med-well 150°-155° well-done 160°-165°.

Prep Time: 40 Minutes

Cook Time: 50 minutes

Servings: 6

Ingredients

Filling:

- 3 cups wild mushrooms (we use chanterelles)
- 3 tbsp butter
- 1 small onion, diced
- 1/2 tsp salt
- 1/2 tsp freshly ground black pepper
- 1/3 cup crème fraîche
- 1/4 tsp fresh thyme
- 3/4 cup gruyere cheese, shredded
- 1 egg, for wash
- Herb Crust
- 2 1/2 cups flour
- 1 tbsp sugar
- 1 tsp salt
- 2 tsp fresh chives, minced

- 1 tbsp fresh thyme, minced
- 1 tbsp flat leaf parsley, minced
- 12 tbsp unsalted butter, cubed and chilled
- 6 tbsp ice water

Instructions

1. In a large mixing bowl, whisk flour, sugar, salt, chives, thyme and parsley in a bowl. Once herbs are coated in flour and evenly dispersed, use a pastry cutter, or a fork to cut butter into flour mixture, forming pea-size crumbles. Add water; work dough until flour and butter are incorporated. Do not over mix. Form the dough into a flat circle and wrap it in plastic wrap. Chill in refrigerator for at least 20 minutes before using.

2. While crust is chilling, make the filling. Using a wet paper towel, "wash" mushrooms. Slice them into ¼ thick pieces. Melt butter in a heavy skillet. Add onions and saute for 3-5 minutes on medium heat. Add the mushrooms and increase heat to medium-high. Cook mushrooms for 5-7 minutes until mushrooms are tender and most of the liquid has evaporated. Season with salt and pepper. Turn heat off and set aside.

3. Preheat oven to 400° F.

4. On a lightly floured surface, roll dough into a 15-inch circle about ¼ inch thick. Carefully transfer to a parchment paper lined baking sheet.

5. Spread the crème fraîche onto the rolled out crust. Starting in the center work your way out, leaving a 2-inch border all around. Using a slotted spoon, scoop the mushroom mixture out of the pan and gently place on top of the crème fraîche. Top with gruyere and sprinkle with fresh thyme. Fold the border up and over the filling, pleating as needed.

6. In a small bowl, whisk the egg with 2 tablespoons water. Using a pastry brush, brush egg wash over the dough rim.

7. Bake the galette for 45-50 minutes. If the crust starts getting too brown, tent with foil. Let cool on a wire rack for 5 minutes before slicing and serving.

Prep Time: 15 Minutes

Cook Time: 20 minutes

Servings: 6

Ingredients

- 4 tablespoons butter
- 2 tablespoons extra-virgin olive oil
- 1 pound mushrooms, thinly sliced, such as crimini or baby bella
- 4 cloves garlic, minced
- 1 cup dry white wine, such as Sauvignon Blanc
- 1 cup chicken or vegetable stock
- 1 cup heavy cream
- ¼ cup freshly grated Parmesan cheese
- 1 pound rigatoni pasta, cooked according to instructions drained
- ¼ cup minced chives
- 2 tablespoons minced flat leaf parsley
- 1/2 teaspoon kosher salt
- 1/4 teaspoon freshly cracked black pepper

Instructions

1. Heat the butter and olive oil in a large saucepan over medium high heat. Once the butter is bubbling, add the mushrooms and cook until golden brown, 5-7 minutes. Add the garlic and cook, stirring, until fragrant, about 2 minutes more.
2. Stir in the wine and simmer until the wine has reduced by slightly more than half.
3. Add the stock and simmer until reduced by half.
4. Slowly stir in the cream and Parmesan until combined. Cook until the sauce comes together and thickens enough to coat the back of a wooden spoon, another 2-3 minutes.
5. Stir in the pasta, chives, parsley, salt and pepper.

Prep Time: 20 Minutes

Cook Time: 15 minutes

Servings: 4

Ingredients

- 1 lb asparagus, trimmed
- 1 1/2 lbs salmon filet, skin on
- 2 Tbsp Extra virgin olive oil
- 3/4 tsp salt
- Blackened Seasoning
- 1 tsp paprika (not smoked)
- 1/8 tsp cayenne
- 1 tsp garlic powder
- 1 tsp onion powder
- 1/2 tsp salt
- 1 tsp dried oregano
- 1 tsp dried thyme
- 1/2 tsp ground ginger
- 1 Tbsp brown sugar

- Cilantro Ginger Sauce
- 1 bunch cilantro, leaves and stems, ends trimmed, about 2 cups packed
- 1 garlic clove, smashed
- 1/4 cup extra-virgin olive oil
- 1 tsp orange zest
- 1/4 cup fresh squeezed orange juice, from 1 orange
- 1/2 tsp honey
- 3/4 tsp kosher salt
- 1 tsp blackened seasoning
- 2 tsp minced fresh ginger

Instructions

1. Preheat oven to 400°F. Prepare a rimmed baking sheet with parchment paper or foil. Place the salmon skin side down on the baking sheet. Pat dry with a paper towel. Place the asparagus on the baking sheet around the salmon.

2. Drizzle the olive oil over the asparagus and a little on the salmon too. Sprinkle the asparagus with the salt and toss them a little to coat.

3. Make the blackened seasoning: In a small bowl, mix all ingredients until fully combined. Reserve 1 teaspoon of

seasoning for the cilantro ginger sauce and sprinkle the remaining over the salmon, rubbing to completely coat it.

4. Place the salmon and asparagus in the oven. Cook until the salmon is tender and the salmon is flaky, about 13-16 minutes depending on the thickness of your salmon and asparagus.

5. Make the cilantro-ginger sauce: Add all ingredients to the base of a high powdered blender or a food processor. Pulse or blend until mostly smooth.

6. Serve the salmon and asparagus drizzled with the cilantro ginger sauce.

21. Green Bean Casserole

Prep Time: 20 Minutes

Cook Time: 30 minutes

Servings: 10

Ingredients

- 2 pounds fresh or frozen green beans
- 2 tablespoons unsalted butter
- 2 tablespoons flour
- 1 teaspoon onion powder
- 1 teaspoon garlic powder
- 1 teaspoon sea salt
- 1/2 teaspoon freshly cracked black pepper
- 1/4 teaspoon ground nutmeg
- 1 teaspoon Dijon mustard
- 1 cup vegetable or chicken stock
- 2 cups half and half
- 1 1/2 cups French fried onions

Instructions

1. Preheat the oven to 375°F.
2. Heat a large pot of salted water to a boil over high heat. Prepare a large bowl of ice water.
3. Add the green beans to the boiling water and cook until nearly tender, about 5 minutes for fresh or 3 minutes for frozen. Drain green beans and transfer them to the ice bath for 2 minutes. Drain green beans again, pat them dry and add them to a 9x13 baking dish.
4. In a large saucepan over medium-high heat, melt the butter. Whisk in the flour, onion powder, garlic powder, salt, pepper, nutmeg and dijon, and cook, whisking occasionally, until fragrant, about 2 minutes.
5. Slowly whisk in the stock until smooth. Slowly whisk in the half and half until combined. Bring the mixture to a simmer over medium heat and cook until thickened, stirring occasionally, about 5 minutes.
6. Pour the sauce over the green beans and toss until fully coated.
7. Bake on center rack until sauce starts to bubble, about 20 minutes. Remove from the oven, toss the green beans and sprinkle with fried onions. Continue to bake on center rack until golden brown, about 10 more minutes.

Prep Time: 15 Minutes

Cook Time: 40 minutes

Servings: 6

Ingredients

- Salisbury Steaks
- 2 large eggs, beaten
- 1/2 cup whole milk
- 3 tablespoons ketchup
- 1 1/2 teaspoon sea salt
- 1 teaspoon Italian seasoning
- 1 teaspoon garlic powder
- 1 teaspoon onion powder
- 1 teaspoons mustard powder
- 1 teaspoons Worcestershire sauce
- 1/4 teaspoon freshly cracked black pepper
- 1 1/2 pounds 90/10 ground beef
- 3/4 cup breadcrumbs
- 1 tablespoon extra-virgin olive or vegetable oil
- Minced fresh parsley leaves, for serving (optional)
- Gravy

- 1 tablespoon extra-virgin olive or vegetable oil
- 1/2 medium yellow onion, thinly sliced
- 10 ounces cremini mushrooms, thinly sliced
- 3 garlic cloves, minced
- 2 tablespoons all-purpose flour
- 1 teaspoon mustard powder
- ¾ teaspoon sea salt
- ¼ teaspoon garlic powder
- ¼ teaspoon onion powder
- 2 tablespoons unsalted butter
- 2 cups beef broth
- 2 teaspoons Worcestershire sauce
- 1 teaspoon better than Bouillon beef base or 1 beef bouillon cube
- Freshly cracked black pepper

Instructions

1. Make the steaks. In a medium bowl, whisk together the eggs, milk, ketchup, salt, Italian seasoning, garlic powder, onion powder, mustard powder, Worcestershire sauce, and black pepper.

2. In a large bowl, combine the ground beef and breadcrumbs. Using your hands, mix gently to combine.

3. Add the egg mixture to the ground beef and again using your hands, gently combine until mixed well. Form the ground beef mixture into 6 oval-shaped patties, about 1-inch thick.

4. Heat the oil in a large skillet over medium heat. Once the oil is glistening, add the patties. Cook without disturbing until browned on the outside but not yet cooked through, about 4 minutes per side. Transfer the patties to a plate.

5. Make the gravy. Heat the olive oil in the same skillet over medium heat. Once the oil is glistening, add the onions and cook, stirring occasionally, until soft and translucent, 6 to 8 minutes. Add the mushrooms and cook, stirring occasionally, until softened, about 5 minutes more. If the pan seems too dry, add ¼ cup of the beef stock. Add the garlic and cook, stirring, until fragrant, about 1 more minute.

6. Add the butter to the pan. Once it is melted, stir in the flour, mustard powder, salt, garlic powder, and onion powder. Slowly stir in the beef broth, Worcestershire, and bouillon.

7. Increase the heat to medium-high and bring the gravy to a boil. Nestle the browned beef patties into the gravy. Cover the skillet and reduce the heat to low. Simmer until the internal temperature of the Salisbury steak patties reaches 160°F on an instant-read thermometer, 10 to 15 minutes.

8. Serve the Salisbury steaks with the gravy spooned over the top. Garnish with minced parsley.

Prep Time: 35 Minutes

Cook Time: 45 minutes

Servings: 10

Ingredients

- 1 pound rigatoni
- 1 pound ground Italian sausage
- 1 pound 90/10 ground beef
- 1 cup diced yellow onion
- 4 garlic cloves, minced
- 1 (24 ounce) jar marinara sauce or homemade
- 1 (24 ounce) can crushed tomatoes
- 1 teaspoon kosher salt
- 1 tablespoon Italian seasoning
- 4 tablespoons salted butter
- 3 cups grated mozzarella cheese
- Minced parsley, for serving

Instructions

1. Preheat the oven to 350°F.

2. Heat a large pot of salted water to a boil over high heat. Add the rigatoni and cook according to the package instructions for al dente. Drain and set aside.

3. Meanwhile, in a large pot or dutch oven, set over medium high heat, cook the sausage, ground beef, onions and garlic, breaking up the meat, until cooked through and onions are softened, about 10 minutes.

4. Add the marinara, crushed tomatoes, salt, Italian seasoning and butter to the meat and cook, stirring often, until butter is melted and sauce is fully combined.

5. Add the rigatoni to the sauce and stir to combine.

6. Transfer the pasta to a 9x13 baked dish. Top with mozzarella, cover and bake for 25 minutes. Uncover and bake for another 10-15 minutes until the cheese is bubbling.

7. Let stand for 5-10 minutes. Top with parsley and serve.

Prep Time: 60 Minutes

Cook Time: 45 minutes

Servings: 6

Ingredients

- 5 cups ½ inch-diced bread cubes from a rustic country loaf, crusts removed
- 2 tablespoons extra-virgin olive oil
- 1 tablespoon unsalted butter
- 2 ounces pancetta, finely diced
- 2 cups thinly sliced leeks, white and light green parts only, washed
- 1 medium yellow onion, diced
- 1 pound cremini mushrooms, trimmed, ¼ inch-sliced
- 1 tablespoon chopped fresh tarragon leaves
- ¼ cup medium or dry sherry
- 2 teaspoons kosher salt
- 1 teaspoon freshly cracked black pepper
- ⅓ cup minced flat leaf parsley
- 4 large eggs
- 1 ½ cups heavy cream

- 1 cup chicken stock
- 6 ounces Gruyère cheese, grated, divided (1 ½ cups)

Instructions

1. Preheat the oven to 350°F with a rack in the center position. Coat a 9x13-inch with olive oil.
2. Spread the bread cubes on a large rimmed baking sheet and bake until lightly browned, 15 minutes.
3. In a large skillet over medium, heat the olive oil and butter, stirring, until melted. Add the pancetta and cook, stirring, until starting to brown, about 5 minutes. Stir in the leeks and onion and cook until the leeks are tender and onion is translucent, 8 to 10 minutes. Stir in the mushrooms, tarragon, sherry, salt and pepper, cook until most of the liquid evaporates, 10 to 12 minutes. Remove from heat and stir in the parsley.
4. In a large mixing bowl, whisk together the eggs, cream, chicken stock and 1 cup of Gruyère. Add the bread cubes and mushroom mixture to the bowl, stirring until combined. Set aside at room temperature for 30 minutes to allow the bread to absorb the liquid. Stir the bread mixture before transferring it to the prepared baking dish

5. Sprinkle with the remaining ½ cup Gruyère and bake until the top is browned and the custard is set, no longer jiggling in the center, 40 to 45 minutes. Serve warm.

6. Adapted from Barefoot Contessa Foolproof by Ina Garten

Prep Time: 45 Minutes

Cook Time: 1hr 15 minutes

Servings: 10

Ingredients

- 16 oz ground Italian sausage, mild
- 1/2 cup (1 stick) butter plus more for baking dish
- 12 cups french bread, (roughly 2 lbs, and day-old, crust cut off, torn or cut into 1-inch pieces)
- 2 cups yellow onions, chopped
- 2 cups celery ¼-inch dice
- 1/2 cup flat-leaf parsley, chopped
- 1 tbsp fresh sage, minced
- 1 tbsp fresh rosemary, minced
- 1 tbsp fresh thyme, chopped
- ¼ tsp nutmeg
- ½ tsp salt
- ½ tsp black pepper, freshly ground
- 2 ½ cups chicken broth, divided
- 2 eggs

Instructions

1. Preheat the oven to 300°. Scatter bread in a single layer on a rimmed baking sheet. Bake, stirring every 15 minutes, until dried out, about 45 minutes. Transfer to a very large bowl.

2. Turn the oven to 350°. Butter a 9x13 baking dish, set aside.

3. Brown the sausage in a large skillet set over medium-high heat. When the sausage is half way browned and crumbled, add the stick of butter onion and celery. Sauté for 5 minutes longer until the sausage is completely browned.

4. Add the onion mixture to the bowl with the bread; add in parsley, sage, rosemary, thyme, nutmeg, salt, and pepper. Toss to evenly disperse the herbs and vegetables with the bread.

5. Drizzle 1 ½ cups broth over the bread mixture and gently toss to combine.

6. Whisk remaining 1 cup broth and eggs in a bowl. Add to the bread mixture; fold gently until thoroughly combined.

7. Transfer to a buttered 9x13 baking dish, cover with foil, and bake for 30 minutes. NOTE: If you are making this recipe a day ahead of time, stop here! Let the stuffing

cool, and place it in the fridge overnight. The next day, bring it out of the fridge about 30 minutes before you're ready to finish baking it.

8. Remove foil, bake until set (no longer jiggly) and top is browned and crispy on top, 45 minutes longer.

26. Herby Rhodes Rolls

Prep Time: 5 Minutes

Cook Time: 20 minutes

Servings: 36

Ingredients

- 1 36 count bag of Rhodes Rolls, or however many you need
- 2 stick butter, melted
- 1 tbsp dried rosemary, crushed in your hand
- 1 tbsp dried oregano
- 1 tbsp dried thyme
- 6 cloves garlic, minced

Instructions

1. In a small saucepan melt butter over low heat and add in herbs and garlic. Cook on low until just melted and very fragrant, careful not to brown.
2. Working with one roll at a time, roll the frozen Rhodes rolls in the herb butter and set in a greased baking pan

about 2" apart. Let the rolls rise 4 to 5 hours, until rolls double in size.

3. Preheat oven to 350°F. Bake for 15-20 minutes, until golden brown.

4. Remove rolls from oven and brush with any remaining melted butter and top with flaky salt. Serve warm.

Prep Time: 15 Minutes

Cook Time: 20 minutes

Servings: 4

Ingredients

- Sandwich
- 8 slices ciabatta bread
- 1/4 cup mayonnaise
- 1/2 cup homemade basil pesto
- 8 oz apple wood bacon, cooked
- 2 cups arugula
- 1 large heirloom tomato, sliced
- 4 eggs

Instructions

1. To assemble the sandwiches, place bread under an oven's broiler for 1 minute to get some nice, brown, toasty color and crunch.

2. On the soft side of one slice of the bread/toast, spread
    1 tablespoon mayonnaise. On the other slice of bread,
    spread 2 tablespoons pesto.
3. Layer on the bacon, arugula, and tomato.
4. Fry eggs to desired yolk runniness. Place one egg on
    each sandwich and enjoy.

Prep Time: 25 Minutes

Cook Time: 35 minutes

Servings: 6

Ingredients

- 1 pound ground beef, 80/20
- 1/2 pound ground pork
- 3/4 cup bread crumbs
- 2 large eggs, beaten
- 3/4 cup whole milk
- 2 tsp sea salt
- 1 tsp Italian seasoning
- 1/4 tsp ground black pepper
- 1 tsp garlic powder
- 1 tsp onion powder
- 1/4 cup ketchup
- 2 Tbsp Brown sugar
- 2 tsp Worcestershire sauce
- 1 tsp water
- ½-3/4 lb broccoli, florets
- ½-3/4 lb baby potatoes, halved

- 2 Tbsp extra virgin olive oil

Instructions

1. Preheat the oven to 350°F.
2. Grease a large rimmed baking sheet, set aside.
3. In a large bowl mix together the ground beef, pork and breadcrumbs until fully combined.
4. In a medium-sized bowl, whisk the eggs together with the milk, 1 1/4 teaspoon salt, Italian seasoning, pepper, garlic powder, and onion powder.
5. Stir the whisked egg mixture, and 3 tablespoons ketchup into the meat, until fully combined. Use a stand mixer for this step if you have one.
6. In a small bowl mix together the remaining 1 tablespoon ketchup, brown sugar, Worcestershire sauce and water until fully combined.
7. Place the broccoli and potatoes on the baking sheet and drizzle with olive oil and remaining 3/4 teaspoon salt. Toss to coat evenly and spread it all out on the baking sheet. Divide the meat into 6 pieces and create an oval about 4" by 3". Nestle them between the broccoli and potatoes.

8. Using a pastry brush, brush the brown sugar sauce over the tops of the meatloaves.

9. Bake in the oven for 30 minutes until the internal temperature of the meatloaf registers 160°F with an instant read thermometer.

Prep Time: 5 Minutes

Cook Time: 20 minutes

Servings: 6

Ingredients

- 6 boneless pork chops, 1-inch thick
- 3/4 cup mayonnaise
- 2 tbsp stone-ground mustard
- 1/4 tsp chili flakes
- 1 tbsp Worcestershire sauce
- 3 garlic cloves, minced
- 1/2 tsp salt
- 1 bunch asparagus, trimmed and cut into 3" pieces
- 2 scallions, thinly sliced, optional

Instructions

1. Preheat oven to 375°F.
2. In a small bowl combine mayonnaise, stone ground mustard, chili flakes, Worcestershire and garlic.

Arrange pork chops on one half of a rimmed baking sheet and coat with mayonnaise mixture.

3. Arrange prepared asparagus on the other half of your baking sheet, and toss it with olive oil and salt.

4. Place baking sheet in oven on center rack and bake for 20 minutes or until pork chops are cooked through.

5. Garnish with scallion.

Prep Time: 15 Minutes

Cook Time: 18 minutes

Servings: 6

Ingredients

- 1 lb large, raw, shrimp, peeled, deveined, tail on
- 1 lb chicken sausage, fully cooked
- 1 lb asparagus, trimmed and cut into 3" pieces
- 2 medium shallots, sliced into wedges
- 1 Tbsp Extra virgin olive oil
- 1 tsp salt
- 2 tsp Old Bay Seasoning
- 1 lemon
- pepper, to taste
- Lemon Garlic Aioli
- 1 cup neutral oil (such as avocado or vegetable)
- 1 egg
- 1 garlic clove, smashed
- zest of one lemon
- 1 Tbsp fresh lemon juice, from 1 lemon
- 1 tsp salt

Instructions

1. To make the aioli, add the oil, egg, garlic, lemon juice and zest and salt to a mason jar. Place hand blender (also known as an immersion blender) at the bottom of the jar and turn it on. In a few seconds you will see the aioli start to form at the bottom. It will quickly begin to emulsify and become thick. Hold the blender at the bottom of the jar for the first few seconds until the oil has been incorporated, then move the blender up slowly until fully combined!

2. Heat oven to 400°F.

3. In a large bowl toss asparagus and shallots in olive oil with 1/2 teaspoon salt and spread on baking sheet along with sausage. Place on center rack and roast for 10 minutes.

4. Remove pan from oven and add shrimp. Season entire sheet pan with remaining salt, freshly ground pepper, old bay seasoning and squeeze the lemon over the top. Gently toss all ingredients on the pan and roast for an additional 6-7 minutes or until sausage is warmed through and shrimp is pink. Serve warm with the aioli. Enjoy!